Holistic Dental Diet

The Comprehensive Guide to Strong Teeth, Healthy Gums and Cavity Prevention

Stacey Ivy Warren D.D.S

Copyright

Copyright © 2024 by Stacey Ivy Warren All rights reserved. No portion of this book, except for brief review, may be reproduced, stored in a retrieval system, or transmitted in any form or by any means—electronic, mechanical, photocopying, recording, or otherwise— without the written permission of the publisher.

MEDICAL DISCLAIMER: The following information is intended for general information purposes only. Individuals should always see their health care provider before administering any suggestions made in this book. Any application of the material set forth in the following pages is at the reader's discretion and is his or her sole responsibility.

Table of Contents

Copyright 1

Table of Contents 2

Introduction 5

Chapter 1 11

The Unnoticeable Toothbrush 11

Chapter 2 18

Your Tooth Tour: Your Teeth Are Alive 18

    True Color Comes from Within 23

    The Gums: Guardians for the Teeth 26

    Super Saliva 29

    External Narrative: Bacteria 31

    Internal Narrative: The unnoticeable Toothbrush 33

    The Endocrine Axis - Hypothalamic-Parotid Gland 35

Chapter 3 41

Potentially Dangerous if Consumed 41

    The Real Deal regarding Mouthwash, Toothpaste, and Toothbrushes 41

    Toothbrushes 55

    Have a Good Time Flossing? 57

    Changing Behaviors 57

    Questionnaires for Potential Dental Patients 59

    Prepping for a Dental Appointment 62

Chapter 4 64

Refined Food Equals Refined Teeth 64

    Consume Food for Your Teeth 65

    Essential Dietary Guidelines 72

    Supplements and Vitamins for Dental Health 74

Chapter 5...**78**

Dental Care for Children **78**

    Feeding the Mouths of Babies 78

Chapter 6...**86**

Braces: Integrated Health or Heavy Metal **86**

    Braces Alter Faces..87

    Teeth Pulling 90

    Be Aware of Your Mouth 92

Chapter 7...**95**

Eight Steps to Self-Dentistry **95**

    Step 1: The Salt-Water Rinse 96

    Step 2: Tongue Scraping 97

    Step 3: Brush the Gums 98

    Step 4: Teeth Polishing 99

    Step 5: Examine the Gum Lines 100

    Step 6: Flossing 101

    Step 7: Final Rinse...101

    Step 8: Extra Gum Care...102

    Review of the Eight Steps 103

Chapter 8...**105**

Botanicals that are Beneficial...**105**

Chapter 9...**117**

Extra Tooth Tips...**117**

Preserving Alkaline Bodies 117
Atomic Mouth Gargle with Iodine 117
Baking Soda 118
Blood Tests 119
Breath 121
Clay 122
Dry Brushing 123
Handling Severe Gum inflammation 123
Healing Herbs 124
Detox for Heavy Metal 125
Homeopathy 126
Salts from Tissue and Cells 128
Hydrogen Peroxide 130
Magnesium Oil Cleansing 131
Therapy with Oil Pulling 131
Ozone Therapy for Dental Health 132
Salt 134
Saunas 134
Thyroid Care 135
Toothaches 136
The Temporomandibular Joints 137
Water 138

Introduction

If, like me, you were brought up in the New World popularly known as **North American** culture and have been instilled with the value of cleaning your teeth and scheduling twice-yearly dental examinations since you were a young child. The skills of brushing and flossing were imparted to you by your parents, assuming they were teaching you these skills. If you had a typical teenage diet, you might have already experienced dental problems like cavities by the time you reached adolescence and became comfortable with handling social situations.

We were not really set up for successful oral care as children, and the reason for this is simple: our parents, and even our dentists, were not very knowledgeable about how to take care of and nourish our teeth and gums. This is something I learned while researching dental self-care, a topic that greatly interests me. We may still have cavities and possibly even require surgical procedures like root canals and extractions even if we followed the recommended regimen of brushing, flossing, and biannual dental checkups. Without complete knowledge of the situation, we tried our best.

You most likely came up with ways to get out of the dentist chair after you were an adult and your parents weren't there to drive you. I did; it felt more comfortable not to be aware of what was happening in my mouth. Maybe my mouth was recoiling from the unusual taste of fluoride, metal, and froth, and my nose was wary of the antiseptic ethers, and I was intuitively revolting against orthodontic contraptions. However, my avoidance resulted in oral entropy, which made a visit to the dentist inevitable wisdom not supporting my disobedience.

I was also raised with the belief that dentists were needed to take care of the mouth and physicians of medicine the body. Thus, like a lot of other people, I thought that the mouth and the body were distinct entities. When I noticed this odd "disconnect" between our conceptions of the mouth and body, I was surprised by how Western dentistry and medicine address symptoms rather than the underlying causes of imbalances in the body. This approach to addressing symptoms leads to an endless round of consultations, prescription drugs, operations, scaling, bridges, crowns, and fillings—none of which ever address or address the fundamental reasons of the imbalance. The statistic that sixty percent of sixty-year-olds having sixty-three percent of their teeth missing, filed, or decaying may be explained by treating the decay rather than treating the causes. Thank goodness, the light emerged, allowing me to emerge from this deeply ingrained cultural mouth-body separation. I started to perceive and comprehend the body's fundamental impulse to realign and rejuvenate, and I realized that the teeth had to be a part of that process.

It's possible that you already know a lot about what dental care strategies work. It's possible that you got your mercury fillings removed. You may be an avid flosser and aware of the risks associated with fluoride exposure. Knowing the value of every tooth as an advocate for excellent oral hygiene who strives for dental care self-sufficiency, you are understandably taken aback when your dentist informs you of receding gums or a cavity.

What happens next? You don't have to ignore your teeth in order to avoid the dentist. You can avoid going to the dentist because you are decay-free and aware of your oral ecosystem, not because you are frightened to go. You can maintain the strength and beauty of your teeth while avoiding dental discomfort with just a little further knowledge. All you need to do is pick up some new habits and a regular maintenance schedule that includes some easy at-home techniques that your dentist from childhood never taught you.

I will walk you through the process of developing new dental care techniques and getting rid of old, inefficient ones on the pages that follow, so you can develop healthier, stronger teeth, gums, saliva, and enamel. I'll give you a tour of your mouth and explain the complex interrelationships between the internal and environmental elements that affect oral health. You will get an understanding of a healthy oral ecology and discover how to eliminate active decay from your mouth using doable techniques that benefit your teeth and your body as a whole. You will wake up with fresh breath and be ready to take on the day when you apply your newfound wisdom. You will also feel your saliva strengthening the gum pockets surrounding each tooth and enameling your teeth. This book will assist you in making well-informed decisions on the long-term health of your oral cavity, even if you still see a dentist sometimes.

Chapter 1

The Unnoticeable Toothbrush

Despite our education to avoid tooth decay through brushing twice a day, flossing, and regular exams, the alarming number of cavities, crowns, root canals, and extracted teeth indicates that we are not getting enough oral care. Dental decay has increased over the past century more than it has in any other, despite the abundance of fluoride treatments, mouthwashes, and periodontal promises.

Dentists and dental colleges generally believe that acids and sugars left on teeth are what cause tooth decay. The International Association of Dental Research convened a symposium in the 1940s that established the norm for this ubiquitous and enduring idea, known as the acidogenic theory. During this crucial meeting, cavities were officially linked to acid erosion, rendering all other systemic theories that had been put out as "fringe." The times are transforming. The field of dentistry is just beginning to recognize the connection between the metabolism of the body as a whole and the mouth. It has been shown by researchers that there are connections between general health and dental health. According to Dr. Reinhard Voll, the originator of electrodermal screening, also known as electroacupuncture, 80 percent of illnesses are linked to dental decay based on his forty years of research. According to his reasoning, any infection that exists in the mouth has an impact on our general health because teeth are linked to every organ and gland through the bloodstream.

Mind Your Mouth

The body's innermost organ, the brain, may be accessed through the mouth, as we now know. The state of the brain is correlated with oral health. The dentist Dr. Ralph Steinman started to doubt the acidogenic explanation of dental disease in 1958. His inspiration came from groundbreaking dental texts published in the 1800s that calculated the amount of lymph circulation within teeth. Steinman's personal experience of the body's interconnection, which included curing his crippling asthma by avoiding processed foods and sweets, piqued my interest. He began to doubt the acidogenic theory's suitability, which holds that teeth are only inactive appendages in a destructive environment and rejects the idea that teeth are essential organs capable of resisting and renewing, as a result of both the dental text and his own experience.

The idea that teeth might have an internal lymph-like fluid serving as a strengthened defense against cavities inspired Steinman to investigate the possibility. He conducted research and created a method that let him see the flow of dentinal fluid in rats by employing a fluorescent dye marker. Steinman's tracking of the dye allowed him to record the startling discovery that teeth are, in fact, inwardly active. Within six minutes of the rat's stomach dye injection, it was visible in the tooth's inner pulp chamber, and an hour later, it was visible in the enamel. Within the teeth, he discovered a continuous, microscopic fluid flow that rises and exits via the tooth from the vicinity of the intestine. In order to prevent gum disease and tooth decay, this dentinal fluid cleans the teeth of toxins, nourishes the mineral matrix of the tooth, and dislodges microbial biofilms from the surfaces of the teeth. Like sap in a tree, it spreads centrifugally outward and upward through the tooth pulp and into the enamel. The end result is that it resembles minuscule sweat beads on the enamel's surface. On the enamel's surface, tiny droplets congregate to create a fluid layer that acts as protection. The fluid volume increases to the location of any enamel break, much like sap does in response to a cut in a tree's bark. It is a nice, flawless procedure. Like bones, teeth are living structures that interact dynamically with the body and mind. As such, they have the ability to regenerate new tissue and last in an environment free from bacteria and acid.

The movement of the flow inside the teeth reverses and becomes centripetal when this dentinal fluid pathway is disrupted, sucking fluids inward from the mouth like a straw. Acids and germs from the mouth are drawn into the teeth by this reverse flow. Acid, fungus, bacteria, and microbes are all actively pulled into the teeth. This reversal of fluid flow causes inflammation in the tooth's pulp chamber, demineralization and oxidative damage, and the start of decay visible through the enamel. Dentinal fluids, when in a healthy flow, supply minerals and nutrients that aid in the ongoing repair and upkeep of the tooth's structure. Salivary enzymes start to break down the structure of teeth when this mechanism is compromised, and bacteria multiply in reaction to the dying tissue.

Steinman was curious as to what causes and controls this fluid. What results in a state of sound flow and what prevents it? To find the source, he teamed up with John Leonora, an endocrinologist. Over the period of forty years, hundreds of effective tests were conducted, and the outcomes verified that an inherent hormone from the hypothalamus controls the dentinal flow within the inner core of our teeth. The secretion that originates from the hypothalamus, a portion of the endocrine system situated in the brain's center, is responsible for controlling dental lymph flow and maintaining the resilience of teeth. When operating as intended, it functions similarly to an invisible toothbrush by reducing the risk of systemic decay, blocking the entry of bacteria into the tooth, and neutralizing acids on the surface of the teeth.

The parotid hormone, which is generated by the parotid gland, is this "switch" that changes the direction of fluid flow. In order to comprehend the complex, living structure of our mouths, let's first examine the internal architecture of the teeth before delving further into the role of the parotid hormone.

Chapter 2

Your Tooth Tour: Your Teeth Are Alive

The most exciting discovery in my research in oral care can be summed up in one sentence: Your teeth are alive! Growing up, I thought teeth were merely dead, solid bones in my mouth, necessary for chewing and biting, set in stone, as it were. I now know that teeth are alive. Like the eyes, the limbs, and the internal organs, they respond to all the same internal factors, such as nutrition, bacteria, and trauma. Living teeth can heal and regenerate. The current condition of your teeth and your mouth can actually evolve. To deeply understand this and put it to work, it is important to understand what teeth, gums, saliva, and bacteria are all about. So, let's start with a quick overview of the internal architecture of the teeth and the mouth.

- enamel
- dentin
- gum
- pulp
- cementum
- periodontal ligament

- crown
- roots

Inside the tooth is the pulp chamber, also known as the root canal, which contains blood vessels, cells, connective tissue, and nerves. This is where nutrients are transported from the bloodstream to the dental fluid. The roots of the teeth connect the teeth to the jawbone and are covered with cementum, a mineralized collagen tissue. There is an opening at the tip of the root that runs through the cementum and connects the tooth to blood flow and the surrounding tissues.

Thousands of small ligaments protrude from the root surface and anchor the tooth to the jawbone. They provide the tooth with a cushion and act as a shock absorber system that allows the tooth to move slightly. If a tooth is extracted and these ligaments are left in place, they are a prime target for infection and commonly cause a cavitation. With an implanted tooth, there are no ligaments attached; a metal screw is drilled into the jawbone to hold the implant and visible crown in place.

Healthy gums provide a natural barrier against the more than four hundred microorganism species trying to enter the circulatory system through the mouth. The epithelium, the skin in the mouth, is only one cell thick and is designed to keep toxins, bacteria, and infection from entering the body. The gums cover the roots and ligaments and hold the teeth upright in their sockets. They contain thousands of microscopic connective filaments that anchor the tooth to the jawbone. The health of these fibers is reflected in the overall health of the gum tissue. These soft oral tissues absorb whatever comes in contact with them with about ninety percent absorption efficiency. The tiniest break or cut in the epithelium allows toxins and bacteria to enter the bloodstream even more quickly.

The outermost layer is the enamel, which is constantly building up and breaking down all day and night. Under a microscope, the enamel looks like a honeycomb. It is primarily composed of a crystal called hydroxyapatite, a crystalline calcium phosphate. When saliva has a pH value of 7, calcium and phosphate flow freely into the tooth enamel to build more crystals to form strong, dense enamel. When saliva is acidic, with pH below 7, the crystals dissolve and become smaller, causing pores to form in the honeycomb pattern. Porous teeth are susceptible to chipping, crumbling, and staining.

Components of the tooth

Dentine is the protective mineralized layer of living tissue that supports the enamel. Dentine is living tissue, and as the diagram shows, the blood supply ends in the pulp chamber. The capillaries in the pulp are fenestrated, allowing a nutrient-rich fluid to diffuse out of the pulp chamber to be taken up by the pump-like action in the odontoblasts, and then out to the dentine. Odontoblasts are connective tissue cells that form the outer surface of the pulp chamber and carry nutrients from the blood into the dentine via the dentinal fluid flow transport mechanism, which is our invisible toothbrush. Inside the dentine, miles of microscopic tubules radiate from the pulp to the dentine-enamel interface. These vital tubules carry the invisible-toothbrush dental fluid that transports nutrients to the rest of the tooth. The pulp tissue contains stem cells that can differentiate into new odontoblasts, if stimulated by decay or damage, to repair the dentine if dentinal lymph flow, parotid hormone, minerals, and fat-soluble vitamins are present.

Dentine is unique among the tissues of the mouth for its production of osteocalcin, a vitamin K-dependent protein that organizes calcium and phosphorus deposits into the bone for mineralization.

True Color Comes from Within

One question that frequently comes up is how to keep our teeth white. Bleaching is not recommended, ever. I can state with absolute certainty that there is no bleaching kit that will do the job safely, be it from the dentist or the drug store. Eventually those treatments will eat away the enamel, and then the teeth will look duller and ultimately be more vulnerable to staining. Furthermore, bleaching can damage the nerve of a tooth and cause gum recession. To have a bright white smile, you have to create the whiteness from the inside out. Instead of approaching it with a cosmetic patch, approach it internally.

Dentine is naturally white. Tooth enamel is actually translucent, like glass. Hard, healthy, and strong enamel will reveal the whiteness of the healthy dentine inside. The health of the dentine is literally reflected in the color of the tooth. So, the best way to whiten your teeth is always from within. Dentine that is fed plenty of nutrients, minerals, and fat-soluble vitamins creates strong, white teeth. In the following chapters, you will learn how to improve the health of your dentine and thus the whiteness of your smile. It is true that tartar and calculus buildup can discolor and create something other than pearly whites. The buildup holds onto color when you enjoy red wine, green smoothies, turmeric, blueberries, and other foods rich in color. This can easily be removed by polishing the teeth with a mixture of baking soda and salt.

In addition to these layers, each tooth also contains blood vessels, craniosacral fluid, and dentinal fluid. These vital fluids connect the teeth to the body's physiological functions. Each tooth relates to different meridian paths of Qi, or life energy as it is understood in traditional Chinese medicine. Qi contains invisible electric lines that run through the teeth, connecting them to the unified Feld of the body.

Just to get an idea of how vast and intricate each tooth is, consider that one molar alone contains more than three hundred yards of tubules. The vast and intricate scale of these tubules is almost impossible to comprehend, and it helps explain why root canals are so problematic. Teeth are a mineral matrix consisting of multiple tissues of varying density and hardness. Once you understand the complex creation of each tooth, it is easy to imagine how much damage can be caused by drilling, fling, root canals, and extractions. It is like putting a chain saw to your teeth.

As an overview, remember this: teeth are more than just bone. The enamel is alive. The dentine is alive. So are the pulp, the blood vessels, the nerves, the saliva, and the gums. They are living things with the ability to regenerate and heal. The inside of our mouths is one whole living organ—a living ecological system. You can see why it's so important to keep the oral ecosystem healthy with all of the components working together.

The Gums: Guardians for the Teeth

A well-made turtleneck sweater will keep you warm, cozy, and protected from the cold. Your gums do the same thing for your teeth. The area where the gum and the tooth meet are called the sulcus, and it is extremely precious. The union of the gum and the tooth is one of the most important areas to protect. It wraps around each tooth like a little turtleneck sweater; however, when there is decay or a buildup along the gum line, bacteria get in, and in response the gum starts pulling away from the tooth. This is what most people know as receding gums. Healthy gum pockets are less than one-tenth of an inch deep, but when the gum pocket starts to pull away from the teeth and the turtleneck no longer fts snugly, the gums sport a crewneck. This enables bacteria to reach a portion of the tooth that has no protective enamel. It also creates sensitivity to food and hot or cold temperatures.

The gums can be slowly worn away so that the crewneck turns into a loose-fitting cowl-neck. When this happens, you end up with exposed molars, and the enamel below the gum line begins to wear away. When we experience symptoms of decay, we usually think it is the tooth that is in trouble. Most of the time, however, it is the gums, because they are the first area to weaken. More teeth are lost to gum disease than to tooth decay.

The gums are a delicate tissue and prone to inflammation as a result of improper brushing, poor nutrition, and other factors that are discussed throughout this book. Mild inflammation of the gums is called gingivitis. Advanced inflammation of the gums is periodontitis. Gum disease like periodontitis has been linked to premature births, irritable bowel syndrome, and heart issues.

The good news is that inflamed gums are one of the easiest issues to cure. Statistics tell us that at least half of the population has periodontal disease, or disease of the tissues that surround the tooth. But what most people don't know is that this can be turned around as quickly as within twenty-four hours, depending on your overall health. Instead of loose, dark, and unhealthy gums, you can have bright pink and healthy gums that do not bleed and are resistant to decay—without surgery. Surgery may take care of the problem temporarily, but many people find that five to ten years after surgery, their gums recede again as they fall back into old ineffective oral hygiene and nutrition habits.

Remember, your gums are alive, and with proper care, they can regenerate. Even if it has been a while since you visited the dentist, your gums are bleeding, and your teeth are sensitive to cold or hot temperatures, with a few changes to your routine the gum tissue will quickly heal.

Super Saliva

Your saliva is extremely important to the function of your mouth. The major salivary glands include the parotid, the submandibular, the sublingual, and the small labial.

One of the superheroes of the mouth, saliva contains chemicals and enzymes that exist solely to take care of the teeth. Healthy teeth exist in a sea of saliva, a sea of saline alkalinity. Imagine that your mouth is a coral reef and your teeth are the coral, surrounded by an ocean of alkaline saliva. It is designed to bathe the teeth all day long in a solution that has a pH of approximately 7—which is exactly what your teeth and gums need. When your teeth are lubricated in saliva, they are at their absolute healthiest, and in this state, they can heal a lot of decay and prevent new decay from occurring.

Depending on the quality of the saliva, it can remineralize or demineralize teeth. It controls bacterial fora in the mouth, prepares food for digestion, and produces vital hormones. It is a saline solution containing enzymes, peptides, minerals, and bicarbonate. Bicarbonate ions are linked to a healthy saliva flow rate, and a higher concentration of bicarbonate ions helps maintain the alkalinity of saliva. If saliva is too acidic, it dissolves the enamel on your teeth and creates an environment that supports bacteria. The longer the mouth remains acidic, the more damage is done to the enamel. Saliva that is too alkaline excretes excess calcium and can create calculus buildup on the teeth.

The key is to allow saliva to do its job effectively. At the onset of oral decay, the saliva jumps into action to coat the tooth with its beautiful healing fluid. At night when we are sleeping, everything slows down, including the activity of the saliva. This explains the common occurrence of "morning breath," because odor-producing bacteria grow faster at night without the normal regulatory saliva. This is particularly true if you are on prescription drugs, if you snore, or if you sleep with your mouth open. Stay well hydrated with Springwater during the day to encourage good saliva production at night.

External Narrative: Bacteria

Your mouth is a warm and inviting incubator. It is the perfect humid home for both beneficial and deleterious bacteria to settle in and grow. If you have a cavity, which is an infection in the tooth, you should think of it as an open wound, a hole in the enamel. If you had an open wound on your hand, you would take care of it by keeping it clean and protected while exposing it to plenty of air circulation. The same is true for healing a wound in your mouth.

A cavity is a symptom of a greater issue in oral health. The acidogenic theory posits that all tooth decay is the result of acid-creating bacteria. Science has demonstrated that bacteria are not the sole cause, but they are one source of decay. Bacteria feed on food that has collected in the mouth, and then they excrete waste of their own. This forms biofilms, or plaque, that builds up on the teeth, the tongue, the cheek tissues, and the gums. Plaque is an ideal nesting area for germs, which can grow into well-organized colonies of germs. These colonies of bacteria constantly form between the teeth and along the edges of the gums and are then sloughed off. These bacteria are also contagious. As the colonies grow, plaque eventually becomes tartar that eventually hardens into calculus. Plaque, tartar, and calculus block the saliva from doing its job: covering the teeth with a protective coating. Without that protective coating, enamel weakens and decay begins.

The first stage of a cavity is known as a carious lesion. This can also be referred to as an enamel lesion, which means that the surface of the enamel has been compromised, indicated by a brown spot on the enamel. The good news is that when the bacteria are removed and the diet is improved, lesions can be halted and healed.

Internal Narrative: The unnoticeable Toothbrush

That is the external story of decay. There is an internal story as well; it's a story that not every dentist knows. Part of the decay process occurs internally, and this relates back to our dental fluid and invisible toothbrush. Our teeth are fed from their roots, like tree roots drawing up nutrients into the tree. These nutrients come only from our diet, hopefully a diet of pure food and water. Diet also plays an important role in the protective power of saliva's alkalinity. We will explore excellent ways to adjust your diet so you can alkalinize your saliva.

Teeth are alive and are programmed to heal themselves, so they know exactly what to do when decay is brewing. Given the right environment, if a cavity starts to form, the dentine reacts by sending odontoblasts to the cavity site, where they start the healing process by laying down a secondary layer of dentine. The saliva also responds to this oral health event, so if you can get your saliva in the right condition, it will help to defend against a full-fledged cavity.

Decay ranges from some little pinpoint cavities here and there all the way to a tooth that's rotted right of at the gum line; you're not going to grow a whole new crown on it. The little ones will heal and can remineralize up to about eight-hundredths of an inch deep. What will happen in a tooth that is severely decayed is that the stump will form up. Instead of being soft and mushy, it develops a leathery consistency. A healed tooth will remain resistant to decay as long as the oral conditions are beneficial.

The Endocrine Axis - Hypothalamic-Parotid Gland

The image illustrates the pathway of the hypothalamic–parotid gland endocrine axis. This is the bodily mechanism that sustains the fluid flow through the tooth. Communication is initiated with chewing when neural endings in the oral mucosa and tongue distinguish nutritive substrates. These substrates activate neural stimuli signaling the hypothalamus. The hypothalamus responds by telling the parotid gland to release a hormonal secretion. This secretion synchronizes the dentinal fluid flux. This parotid hormone is involved in the formation of dentine and regulates the direction of the flow of dental fluid.

The parotid gland is the largest salivary gland, sitting adjacent to the inner ear. In front of the gland is the jawbone and the masseter muscle. The deep surface of the gland lies alongside the back of the throat near the tonsils. When the parotid gland hormone is produced in adequate amounts, fluid flows into the teeth and delivers essential nutrients for optimal oral health. When parotid gland hormone production is adversely affected, the fluid flow reverses.

Dr. Ralph Steinman identified several suppressors that reverse dentinal lymph. One of the suppressors of dentinal flow is dietary sugar, or sucrose. In the absence of a sugary and carbohydrate-laden diet, the dentinal fluid flows like sap into the tooth. In the presence of a high-sugar, high-carbohydrate diet that includes bread, cereal, pasta, rice, and pastries, no flow occurs. Insulin is one of the primary influencers of the parotid gland. Foods that elevate blood insulin levels, such as refined carbohydrates and sugars, will affect the direction of fluid flow in the teeth. Sugar raises insulin levels and inhibits the hypothalamus from functioning properly. Daily high blood sugar levels suppress dentinal flow. The endocrine axis responds immediately when there is a reduction of dietary sugar to normal blood sugar levels.

Contrary to the acidogenic theory, sugar on the surface of the tooth is not the initiating factor of decay. Some dentists may approve of sugar and carbonated drinks—maybe that is why some pediatric dentists hand out lollipops—as long as you brush your teeth after. The teeth can actually handle sugar sitting on their surfaces. Dental decay is a systemic disease caused by sugars and processed carbohydrates suppressing the endocrine system and switching the signaling messenger to the endocrine system. It is not because you have a piece of food sitting on a tooth.

Processed foods, additives, and deficiencies in dietary nutrients also reverse the dentinal fix. Most of the "flow-in" foods are refined foods.... About the age of two or three years, the permanent teeth are forming within the jawbone. If there is a deficiency of vitamins C, D, or A during calcification [when the teeth are forming], a tooth less resistant to decay will be produced.

Real vitamins and minerals are needed to synthesize new tooth tissue and maintain the body's electrochemistry. Deficiencies in minerals signal the body to take minerals from the teeth and bones for other organs. The nutritive composition of the diet is vital for the secretion of parotid hormone because it is activated through the molecular matter of phytonutrients. In studies by Steinman, the addition of copper, iron, and manganese to a sugar-producing diet almost abolished the decay rate. Intake of phosphorus alone reduced the decay rate by eighty-six percent. Phosphorus also prevented the atrophy and shrinking of the parotid gland associated with the ingestion of sugar.

There are a variety of other factors that can affect dental flow. Stress, with its production of cortisol, along with peak hormonal times in a person's life can be detrimental to the hormonal cascade and hinder the dentinal fluid flow. Hormonal shifts, such as low thyroid activity, pregnancy, the teenage years, and growth spurts in children can affect dentinal flow and make teeth susceptible to decay. Lack of exercise and lymph stagnation also affect the hypothalamic–parotid endocrine axis. Medication, oral care chemicals, antibiotics, and fluoride systemically suppress the hypothalamus and reverse parotid activity.

Much about our hormonal secretions remains a mystery. We do know that the glands secrete the finest of lubricants, orchestrating communication throughout the body. And even though our glands are physically small, they have an enormous capacity to store toxins: the thyroid gland mops up most radiation, and the pineal gland accumulates the most fluoride. The parotid gland can respond to cell-phone radiation with tumors, while fluoride suppresses its hormonal secretion. Yes, that's the same fluoride you find in your toothpaste.

Chapter 3

Potentially Dangerous if Consumed

The Real Deal regarding Mouthwash, Toothpaste, and Toothbrushes

Growing up, brushing your teeth with toothpaste was a common practice that was thought to be one of the healthy habits needed to keep your mouth clean and prevent cavities. It's possible that you've heard the advice to maintain good tooth health by brushing, flossing, and seeing the dentist twice a year. But despite their good intentions, a lot of people found that they were still experiencing dental issues like cavities, bleeding gums, bad breath, and more.

Why is the prevalence of cavities at an all-time rise if toothpaste is our teeth's magical cleaner? Furthermore, why do the majority of toothpaste manufacturers include a large caution sign that says, "may be harmful if swallowed"?

You don't want the kinds of chemicals found in commercial toothpastes in your mouth. These artificial substances are more suited for industrial use than for maintaining dental health or cleaning the body's sensitive tissues. I switched to toothpastes from the health food shop after learning about these chemical compounds, only to discover later that these too contained artificial and dangerous substances. Additionally, I observed that in cases where a product did include herbal extracts, the levels of the extracts were insufficient to effectively benefit the oral ecology.

These substances may be detrimental to our health when brushed on. Because anything in the mouth has direct access to the bloodstream, anything we put in our mouths gets absorbed into the body through the mucous membranes in our mouths. This is particularly true if we have bleeding gums. The moist tissues of the skin wall, or epithelium, inside the mouth are only one cell thick. These artificial compounds have the potential to degrade collagen, interfere with hormones, harm the sensitive epithelium, disrupt intestinal microbiota, and ultimately promote ill health. The common ingredients in toothpaste that can be dangerous to ingest are listed below to help you make informed decisions about what you put into your body.

- **Fluoride:** Tooth decay is not brought on by a lack of fluoride, despite insane marketing claims. Fluoride is listed as having "substantial evidence of neurotoxicity" by the US Environmental Protection Agency. It seems that fluoride tampers with vital physiological chemistry, causing gum damage, collagen formation disruption, and decreased enzyme performance. The body builds up fluoride, particularly in the pineal gland, which causes IQ declines, deposits linked to Alzheimer's disease in the brain, early puberty, and a host of other negative effects.

- **Propylene glycol:** Propylene glycol, or PG, is commonly used as antifreeze and to deice airplanes. It is present in certain kinds of toothpaste. Oil refining is the process that yields propylene from fossil fuels. While not as harmful as its relative ethylene glycol, PG can cause irritation to the skin and mucous membranes, raising the body's acidity to a point where metabolic acidosis results. Despite toothpaste's tiny amount of PG, its frequent daily use raises the possibility of negative effects.

- **FD&C color pigments:** In dental goods, dyes and pigments are harmful and have no health benefit. Children have been reported to become hyperactive for twenty years due to carbon deposits, laboratory-derived colors, and coal tar, all of which are known to be possible allergens. Heavy metals that can build up in the body are included in many of the food, drug, and cosmetic (FD&C) coloring additives that the US Food and Drug Administration (FDA) has allowed.

- **Triclosan:** This licensed insecticide, which is bio persistent, devastates delicate aquatic ecosystems. Additionally, the FDA has approved its usage as an antibacterial ingredient in toothpaste to help prevent gingivitis. The FDA is currently conducting additional assessment of it because of recent research indicating that it might change hormone control. According to a study released by the National Academy of Sciences, "triclosan potently impairs muscle functions." In a sample of 1,571 people, the U.S. Centers for Disease Control and Prevention (CDC) discovered triclosan in the urine of 75% of them. Biologists are beginning to worry about the antibacterial qualities of triclosan. Experimental evidence points to a connection between antimicrobial medication resistance and exposure. Furthermore, triclosan has unfavorable spillover effects on the environment. It adheres to sediments in rivers, lakes, and streams, building up over time and endangering aquatic life.

- **Artificial sweeteners:** Typically, xylitol, sorbitol, and saccharin are added to toothpaste to enhance its flavor. In the 70's, saccharin, a sugar substitute derived from petroleum, was connected to cancer. Reducing glucose yields sorbitol, which is a nutritional waste product. Many fruits and vegetables contain xylitol, which is also made from corncobs and hardwood trees for industrial applications. Since neither sorbitol nor xylitol is entirely absorbed, ingesting them can result in a variety of gastrointestinal issues, particularly in young children: diarrhea, bloating, and abdominal pain. Certain toothpaste manufacturers assert that xylitol is good for gums and teeth because it neutralizes saliva, kills germs, and promotes tooth remineralization. Given that there was inconclusive evidence of this in two clinical trials, these claims are somewhat deceptive.

- **Ethanol:** Getting a large bottle of mouthwash is one of the first things individuals do when they discover they have gum or breath issues. Known to cause oral cancer, you may be surprised to learn that ethanol is the primary ingredient in most mouthwashes. Known to be the cause of over 30,000 occurrences of mouth cancer annually, isopropyl alcohols and ethanol (grain alcohol) are highly irritating and drying solvents derived from propylene, a petroleum byproduct.

- **Detergents and surfactants:** Added to toothpastes to provide a clean, frothy brushing experience, what toothpaste would be complete without detergents and surfactants? In addition to being known skin irritants, surfactants, such as sodium laureth sulfate (SLES), ammonium laureth sulfate (ALES), sodium lauryl sulfate (SLS), and ammonium lauryl sulfate (ALS), are also probable carcinogens and gene mutagens. SLS is known to cause bleeding gums and to disrupt the skin's natural barrier. Additionally, it increases skin permeability by around a hundredfold, which makes it possible for additional substances to permeate.

- **Trisodium phosphate:** Trisodium phosphate (TSP) was commonly used in home cleaners and detergents until the 60's, when scientists discovered that it caused an over bloom of algae in our lakes and rivers. As a result, product manufacturers were under pressure to remove phosphates from their products. Even now, home improvement stores still carry it as a potent cleanser and degreaser.

  TSP can damage skin because of its extremely alkaline pH of 12. It neutralizes extremely acidic conditions produced by carbomers and is used as a cleaning in toothpaste. Since artificial sweeteners in toothpastes are converted into lactic acid, TSP consumption lowers lactic acid buildup, which may be significant. Trisodium phosphate can eventually result in gum bleeding, tumor lesions, and nerve inflammation. It could damage the liver as well.

- **Glycerin:** This smooth, transparent gel is a popular, low-cost filler and carrier for the low-concentration compounds that are identified as active components. Glycerin is produced by continually processing, bleaching, and deodorizing a mixture of dry vegetables, which gives the substance a thick consistency akin to molasses. Glycerin covers the teeth and prevents saliva from performing its main function of restoring enamel mineralization.

- **Calcium:** Toothpaste contains calcium carbonate for various alleged purposes. It is an abrasive cleaning solution that aids in the plaque and tartar removal process. It works as a desensitizing agent to numb teeth that are susceptible to temperature fluctuations. Moreover, producers contend that calcium carbonate remineralizes the dentine and enamel from the outside of the tooth, based on scant clinical evidence. Not water soluble or readily accessible, calcium carbonate is mostly found in eggshells, seashells, limestone, chalk, marble, and other types of stone. When consumed, it can lead to calcifications, kidney stones, hypocalcemia, and joint issues.

- **Flavorings:** We are all familiar with the marketing promise of "minty fresh" from advertising. In order to mask the overpowering, disagreeable taste of detergents like SLS in toothpaste, flavorings are added to oral goods. The majority of goods include artificial cinnamon (cinnamaldehyde) or mint (menthol). Instead of being produced by a plant, these artificial derivatives are created in a beaker. For instance, benzaldehyde, acetaldehyde (which may be carcinogenic), sodium hydroxide (lye), calcium hydroxide (hydrated lime), hydrochloric acid, or sodium ethylate (a corrosive) can all be condensed to produce cinnamon aldehyde. Tastes good! True cinnamon is derived from the essential oils found in cinnamon bark, while minty-fresh peppermint is created from the plant's oils. The mouth and body can benefit from the antibacterial and regenerating properties included in these genuine essences.

- **Carbomer:** One of the byproducts of the manufacture of gasoline is acrylic acid, which is polymerized here. This light-colored, fluffy powder is soluble in water and can be utilized to stabilize and thicken liquid ingredients into a paste, preventing it from separating. Just to appeal to consumers' perceptions of what a tooth cleaner's texture should be, carbomer is incorporated.

Due to the extreme acidity of these polymers, it takes yet another chemical—which might not be mentioned on the label—to neutralize them sufficiently to prevent burns to the lips. Triethanolamine (TEA), sodium hydroxide, and tetrasodium EDTA are examples of potential neutralizers.

- **Carrageenan:** Given that it comes from red seaweed, which sounds natural and healthy, this sticky, gel-like material is frequently overlooked. Scientific investigations conducted recently have found a link between carrageenan and immune system problems, colorectal cancer, and unsettled stomachs.

Hopefully, toothpaste isn't being gulped down by anyone. Oral ecology is not optimally created by chemicals that foam in your mouth. Anything that cannot be eaten should not be placed within, outside, or around the body.

The body's reaction to bacteria entering the mouth is bleeding gums, which is one of the most prevalent illnesses in North America. Due to its prevalence, many choose to overlook it and blame sensitive teeth for it. We've been led to believe by the advertising industry that purchasing a solution designed specifically for sensitive teeth will take care of this discomfort. After purchasing the particular brand of toothpaste, people report that their symptoms are lessened. But the symptoms are just being covered up because these toothpastes numb the mouth, not the painful teeth or the bleeding, receding gums. Anything in the mouth will have instant access to the bloodstream if you have bleeding gums, which are really caused by some of the surfactants in toothpaste.

Giving up all commercial dental products and substituting them with baking soda, salt, a dry toothbrush, and plant treatments that can start the healing process is one of the most crucial parts of effective dental self-care.

Toothbrushes

Now let's discuss toothbrushes. It's possible that your toothbrush become fat after a few months of use. The majority of individuals see this as an indication that it's time to change their toothbrush. Actually, it's telling you something completely different: when you brush, you're applying far too much pressure. You want to brush so sparingly that, instead of your toothbrush looking like a squashed version of itself after six months, it appears exactly like it did when you first bought it.

I advise using both manual and electric toothbrushes. For the past ten years, I have been using an ionic light-activated toothbrush, which is a manual toothbrush that ionizes saliva using light. By exposing you to areas of your mouth you were unaware you could reach, electric toothbrushes are an excellent tool for teaching you how to modify your brushing habits. I find that there is not much of a difference between the premium and inexpensive models. Choose an electric toothbrush with a circular head if you choose to buy one so that you can reach the challenging areas behind the back and front teeth. Always use a soft-headed toothbrush, both electric and manual.

Have a Good Time Flossing?

It's fantastic if you floss every day. It is much better if you use botanical oils for your floss. A single drop of botanical oil can change the process of flossing since it can reach the bacteria in the microscopic gaps between teeth that are too small for floss. After the food is removed by the floss, the germs and interdental plaque are eliminated by the essential oils' potent plant molecules.

Your gums can bleed a little if you haven't had any flossed in a while. If you floss two or three times a day for two or three days, especially with the use of botanical oils, this will clear up. You should observe improvement in a few days if you treat a single tooth that is bothering you and you take additional care of it.

Changing Behaviors

As many of us find taking care of our teeth on a daily basis to be tedious, we often brush and floss automatically. Your everyday rituals will seem more refreshed if you practice mindfulness, and brushing your teeth is a fantastic place to start. Consider brushing anyplace rather than at the bathroom sink with the faucet running and a lump of toothpaste on a wet toothbrush before scrubbing vigorously for twenty seconds. You can brush while sitting at your desk, taking a bath or shower, or even outside in the sun. You'll be shocked at how much more awareness you develop when you shift your location. My favorite spot to clean my teeth is by the seaside, where the sunlight activates my ionic toothbrush. I love to do this whenever I can.

Using a dry toothbrush is preferable to a wet one. More bacteria and plaque can be eliminated from your teeth by utilizing a dry toothbrush and thorough cleaning instead of a wet brush and ordinary toothpaste. Try adding a tiny bit of baking soda to your brush if you'd like. Because saliva and baking soda share comparable biochemical properties, baking soda is a fantastic oral hygiene aid that is also harmonious and congruent with the oral environment. Furthermore, saliva needs something alkaline, which it is. Even better, use a dry brush with a drop of botanical oil added to it to gain antifungal, antiviral, antibacterial, and lipophilic benefits that will reach the gums.

Brushing your teeth immediately after a meal is not the best idea. The saliva won't have time to adjust to its slightly alkaline pH 7 level if you brush too soon after eating. If you would like to, you can rinse with salt water to neutralize the saliva once again.

Questionnaires for Potential Dental Patients

Encouraging you to have a healthy relationship with your teeth and a dentist is my aim. Beyond veneers and teeth whitening, a potential dentist's website should provide useful information. Asking about the specifics of dentistry is helpful when you give the dental office a call. Asking your dentist, the following questions before accepting an appointment can help you make an informed choice.

1. Are water filters used that remove pollutants and bacteria from tap water? As germs can accumulate in water lines, the water you use to rinse your mouth could be tainted with dangerous bacteria.

2. Do they do patient-by-patient biocompatible testing to ensure material compatibility with dental implants? To determine which dental materials your body can tolerate, the dentist can do a blood test. Approximately 60% of dental materials have immune-suppressive properties.

3. Do they clean parts of the mouth, receding gums, and recently filled teeth with ozone or lasers?

4. Do they make use of microscopes with phase contrast? They may assess the

gums' condition well in advance of periodontal disease by extracting germs from the gum line thanks to these microscopes.

5. Is it a mercury-free dental practice?

6. Do they employ digital radiography? You are exposed to 90% less radiation using digital than you would with traditional X-ray machines.

7. Regarding root canals, what is their position?

8. Regarding sealants, what is their position?

9. What is their position on fluoride?

10. Do they develop a nutrition plan for patients?

11. Are intraoral cameras used by them? You and the dentist may examine your mouth together thanks to intraoral cameras, which project an image of your mouth onto a screen.

12. Does the dentist apply a new inlay or crown using a laser? Strong laser bonding eliminates the need for harmful dental cements.

13. Are IV infusions of vitamin C available for use during procedures?

14. When doing dental restorations, does the dentist use a brand-new drill bur?

15. Exists a comprehensive procedure for eliminating amalgam fillings?

Prepping for a Dental Appointment

Even though you clean your teeth well every day, you should still see that amazing new biological dentist you found if your teeth have been neglected for a time or if you have had dental work done in the past that is no longer desirable, such a mercury filling.

Did you know that because blood is likely to be contaminated with bacteria, donating blood is prohibited for 48 hours following dental cleanings? Expert dental cleanings eliminate tartar buildup on teeth, but they are unable to prevent germs that thrive on acid from growing again. Additionally, cleanings don't protect or strengthen teeth. Following a thorough scaling by a hygienist, mouth bacteria become loose and enter the bloodstream, taxing the body's defenses. Systemic inflammation is one of the outcomes of the body's response to this imagined attack, which involves the release of white blood cells to fight the invasive bacteria. Furthermore, a lot of dangerous germs survive in saliva and return to the bloodstream and teeth.

Chapter 4

Refined Food Equals Refined Teeth

The secrets to optimal dental health include eating genuine foods, balancing hormones, getting appropriate minerals from your diet, and allowing proper fluid circulation between your teeth. Our meals have a direct impact on our oral health and vigor. When we nourish the health of our teeth with extremely nutritious foods and clear water, we internally keep healthy mouths.

Processed food is commonplace in our industrialized day. Frozen dinners, sugary snacks, soda pop, dyes, chemicals, and preservatives are all quite popular foods for a lot of people. Fortunately, eating whole, unprocessed foods, pastured foods, wild foods, and superfoods is becoming more and more popular. As we shall see, the foods we eat can either cause or cure cavities, thus this is a positive step.

The medical professionals Edward and May Mellanby, who identified that rickets is caused by a vitamin D deficiency, also investigated the nutritional elements influencing tooth development. The results of their study demonstrated that teeth respond to dental caries by sending odontoblasts to the damaged tissue in order to heal the enamel and dentine.

Regardless of the condition of the tooth's original structure, May Mellanby's research showed that odontoblasts could create a strong, thick layer of secondary dentine when fed a diet rich in phosphorus, vitamin D, and the calcium-forming elements magnesium and silica.

Consume Food for Your Teeth

A really tooth-healthy diet consists of foods abundant in minerals and fat-soluble vitamins E, D3, A, and K2, in addition to whole meals and variety. The body also need hydrochloric acid, plenty of digestive enzymes, and adequate intestinal function for optimal nutritional absorption.

A repository of fat-soluble nutrients that the animals gain from their diet is their body fat when cows, pigs, sheep, and chickens are permitted to consume their natural diets in the pasture. Some of the vitamins and minerals that the animal has stored are consumed when we eat the fat from its meat, organs, eggs, or dairy products. Due to the animals' restricted, non-species-specific, and nutrient-depleted diets, the meat and other easily accessible products derived from factory-raised animals lack adequate levels of these essential elements.

Meat and dairy products include vitamin K2, which is different from the vitamin K that we obtain from eating greens like spinach and kale. Rich in vitamins, pasture-fed butter, egg yolks, and cheeses have deep orange and gold hues. K2 is essential for the formation of bones because it transports dietary calcium to the right places and eliminates excess calcium from tissues. Intestinal fora are also the source of vitamin K2. Fermented foods such as natto (fermented soybeans), sauerkraut, kimchi, and aged Gouda cheese are excellent weekly supplies of this vitamin.

Water-soluble beta-carotene is the form of vitamin A that is obtained from vegetables like carrots. Meat and dairy products raised on pasture have retinol, a vitamin A, which has a distinct biological function than beta-carotene. For good health, both types are essential: retinol is necessary for strong bones, eyes, and skin, while beta-carotene is a potent antioxidant. By preventing free radical damage to the process of creating bones, fat-soluble vitamin E also supports bone health.

For optimal calcium use and for the assimilation of both calcium and proteins, our bodies and bones also require vitamin D and vitamin A. A lack of vitamin D significantly impairs bone formation and maintenance. By exposing our skin to the sun for ten to fifteen minutes each day, we may produce our own vitamin D. In mild winter climates as well as the summer, this is a simple task. Eating natural foods is an important way to enhance your vitamin D consumption during the cold and cloudy seasons. Fish liver oils, particularly cod liver oil, eggs, organ meats, and fish are excellent sources of biologically accessible vitamin D3.

The conventional Western diet is lacking in silica, phosphorus, and magnesium, three minerals that are essential for strong bones. However, these minerals were abundant in ancient periods and indigenous peoples' diets, shielding them from dental disease. Meat from animals kept on pastures is a good supply of silica and phosphorus, which are essential for healthy bones, the jaw, and tooth development. Pasture grasses are a rich source of these nutrients. My favorite food group, chocolate, has a high phosphorus and magnesium content. Eat chocolate as raw and rich as possible, without added sugar, preservatives, or other superfluous ingredients.

For best health, consumption of processed foods deficient in nutrients must be drastically decreased or stopped. Grains, beans, seeds, and nuts contain the antinutrient phytic acid; to avoid this, grow them organically and soak or ferment them before consuming. Mineral absorption is impeded by phytic acid. Phosphorus is bound securely and cannot be absorbed by the body. Inhibiting enzymes required for food digestion, it can also bind to and prevent iron, calcium, zinc, and other elements from the body. Before eating, our sage predecessors in many ancient societies frequently stone-ground, steeped, and fermented grains, nuts, beans, and seeds. Compared to crushed grains, whole grains contain higher phytic acid. Fermenting and grinding stones is a lost craft. Cereals and grains that are ready for the market are usually rancid and undergo bromine processing. Compared to foods cultivated organically, commercially manufactured foods grown with synthetic phosphate fertilizers have higher levels of phytic acid.

Dietary sugar left on the surface of teeth is not the cause of tooth decay. The bacteria in a petri dish will really refuse to ingest sugar if it is added. Sugar in the diet that reduces nutrition, not sugar coming into contact with teeth, is what causes decay. Furthermore, sugar makes the mouth and digestive system more acidic, which is the opposite of what a healthy mouth and salivary system require.

Dr. Weston A. Price has conducted some of the best research on the connection between dental health and processed foods. While serving as president of the American Dental Association in the 20's, he traveled to several cultures where people continued to follow their traditional diets. These cultural groups were following the same customary diets that their ancestors had been following for centuries; they had not been conquered by Europeans and had not been introduced to white bread, white sugar, or chemicals. Price examined their teeth, jaws, and face structure, as well as the jaws of nearby bones. He discovered that there were remarkably few cavities before the 19th century—roughly one cavity for every 1,000 skulls. The statistics of today are the exact opposite of this.

The final word!!! Tooth decay can result from any processed food. The science is straightforward and can be encapsulated in a single sentence: refined and processed meals interfere with the endocrine system and digestion, changing the way nutrients reach the teeth. When nourishment is lacking and the internal ecology has collapsed, coupled with a few generations of malnourished relatives, it is not good for your teeth and gums.

The mouth's tissues are made to be nourished inside. This indicates that the greatest way to be healthy is to avoid processed foods, white sugar, white flour, fizzy drinks, saccharine, high-fructose corn syrup, and convenience store goods altogether—zero.

Essential Dietary Guidelines

The following is an overview of the dietary recommendations derived from the previously mentioned studies:

- To get rid of and evolve phytic acid, all grains, beans, and nuts need to be soaked and fermented.

- Get rid of wheat.

- Consume complete, fresh foods.

- Consume no processed food at all.

- Consume organic produce that has been grown in soil that is high in minerals.

- Consume herbs high in minerals, like nettles and horsetail, blended into smoothies and drinks.

- Take pills containing vitamin D3 or get enough sunlight.

- Consume a range of organ meats because they are high in minerals and vitamins. You can substitute high-quality desiccated glandular supplements if you're not a fan of organ meats.

- Use only virgin olive oil, coconut oil, or ghee from grass-fed cows while cooking.

- Steer clear of any vegetable oils, including corn and soy, and their polyunsaturated fatty acids (PUFAs). Use hemp, pumpkin, and raw organic chia oils to dress salads.

- Vegetarians and vegans must make sure they get adequate amounts of fat-soluble vitamins K2, D3, and A.

- To treat cavities, add fermented cod liver oil to food.

- Consume grass-fed butter or unpasteurized ghee, or take pills containing vitamin K2.

- Wild or organic animal products are the greatest, and raw organic dairy products from cows raised on pasture completed on only grass are also the best.

- Consume a large amount of clean water.

Supplements and Vitamins for Dental Health

Seek for high-quality, naturally sourced vitamins and supplements devoid of excipients like magnesium stearate.

Every cell in the body contains the fatty acid known as (R)-alpha lipoic acid (RALA). It is also a dual-purpose metabolic antioxidant that may neutralize free radicals in blood, lipids, and water. It is a lipophilic and hydrophilic molecule. RALA generates energy for the mitochondria at the cellular level. It increases and recycles glutathione, vitamin C, and vitamin E, among other antioxidants.

The nonessential amino acid cysteine has a derivative and bioavailable form called N-acetyl-L-cysteine (NAC). Glutathione levels are raised by NAC, which is also a very powerful nutritional supplement. According to its antidotal spectrum, even vitamin C cannot equal its detoxifying agent properties.

The most bioavailable kind of vitamin C, found in Lypo-Spheric brand, increases glutathione levels and preserves collagen and blood vessels. Consume amla (Indian gooseberries) and Camu

Camu berries, two organic superfoods that naturally contain vitamin C.

The dietary minerals phosphorus, magnesium, and silica, in addition to the vitamins D3 and K2, help the body produce calcium. Nettles, chia seeds, horsetail herb, leafy greens, and spirulina are excellent sources. A common ingredient in eggshells, seashells, limestone, chalk, marble, and other types of stone, calcium carbonate is neither soluble in water or bioavailable, and consuming it can lead to calcifications, kidney stones, hypocalcemia, and joint issues. Steer clear of calcium carbonate supplements.

Gum tissue and the bone matrix can be restored by the powerful antioxidant coenzyme Q10 in ubiquinol form. It might also cause saliva to produce more.

The primary source of fat-soluble vitamin D3, which is produced by sunlight exposure on human skin, is a steroidal precursor hormone rather than a vitamin. Depending on your skin type and the amount of sun exposure where you live, you might need to take IU supplements or natural food sources in amounts of 5,000 or 10,000 per day.

Immune system function depends on glutathione (GSH), an intracellular antioxidant and tripeptide. Glutathione is a substance found in every cell on Earth. It is well renowned for its capacity to shield and cleanse the body.

While leafy green vegetables provide vitamin K1, animal fat has powerful amounts of fat-soluble vitamin K2. Additionally, there are vitamin K2 pills and liquid forms that are produced from fermented soybean natto.

Chapter 5

Dental Care for Children

Even though we are all grown up, it is never too late to learn, and it is actually a perfect time to teach our children about dental health. When our children are young, we have an opportunity to share ideas about the body's ability to regenerate and implement ideal dietary and oral care practices. Even when children, or teenagers, for that matter, do brush their teeth, are they doing a thorough job? Is their brushing completely effective in clearing away all the plaque? It's unlikely.

Feeding the Mouths of Babies

Beyond brushing, the internal factors that nourish the teeth are so important: eating real foods, hormonal balance, minerals, fat-soluble vitamins, and healthy fluid exchange through the teeth. Stress, processed foods, and inadequate nutrition negatively affect dental fluid flow.

Nutrition is also a significant factor that influences the development of the entire mouth, not just the teeth, and it should include a healthy prenatal diet, breast-feeding, and raising children on real, unprocessed foods. Always provide whole foods, and examine the quality and quantity of vitamins and minerals your child is getting.

Our oral ecology begins before we're born. Babies are generally born without teeth, yet their teeth are already forming. In fact, a baby's teeth begin forming in utero, so certainly preconception and prenatal nutrition are important. Ensure that the fat-soluble vitamins such as A, D3, and K2 are part of your daily nutrition. Vitamin K2 is as important as folic acid for pregnant women. Vitamins K2 and D aid in the development of the bones, including the facial form of the developing fetus. Eating two eggs from grass-fed chickens or a teaspoon or so of ghee from pasture-fed cows are delicious sources of both. You can make sure that you provide the minerals needed for bone development by steeping horsetail, nettles, and oat straw in nearly boiling water. This makes an herbal tea that is full of silica and phosphorus. Add a few drops of ginger essential oil or dried ground ginger to the tea to help settle morning sickness.

Breast-feeding is the best thing that you can do for your baby's health. It is the best means of providing the highest level of nutrition to a baby, and that is of prime importance in your baby's facial and oral development. Only a varied, wholesome, and colorful diet can supply all of the nutrients needed for the complex process that builds and maintains the integrity of our bones. While it is possible to obtain the nutrient requirements as a vegetarian or vegan, it is much simpler to do it with wild fish or pasture-raised meat and dairy in the diet. Mothers who are breast-feeding, take care: you must get large quantities of nutrient-dense food and fresh water to nourish yourself and your child. It is a perfect process; as the baby grows, substances in the breast milk actually evolve to meet the nutritional requirements of the child's changing needs. The act of breast-feeding may also be formative in the proper development of the jaw. Each time we swallow, the tongue pushes upward and fattens in the roof of the mouth. The force of this motion may shape the jaws. Breast-fed babies are fed longer and more frequently, and thus the baby does more swallowing. As the child grows, the top jaw forms around the shape of the tongue, resulting in a broad facial structure with sufficient room to house evenly placed teeth. Tooth decay in babies and toddlers is never caused by breast-feeding. Children grow rapidly in their sleep, and nighttime nursing, which has been done since the beginning of time, has never caused a cavity.

With a new baby, you have a golden opportunity to celebrate a healthy, balanced human being, and a good place to start is with purity in the diet. If you never introduce your child to highly processed foods and junk food, the odds are excellent that he or she will not develop a taste for them. My recommendation is to offer no processed foods whatsoever, including formula and processed juices —even apple juice from a health-food store. The best thing for your baby to drink is pure spring water and breast milk. Certain herbal teas sipped at room temperature, like chamomile and nettle, are also a lovely option. As the child grows and starts eating more solid foods, you will need to include plenty of food rich in fat-soluble vitamins and minerals. As the teeth begin to come in, even though it is too early to brush, you can still take care of them by wiping each tooth with a cloth just to make sure that it is clear of any food or acidic buildup.

Cavities in children were a rare occurrence. Today, one of the biggest health concerns in North America and Europe affecting little ones more than any other age group is dental decay, or early childhood caries (ECC). There is a common misconception that it is normal for kids to have cavities. Children are young, vital, and, of course, growing, so childhood cavities are not an issue of degenerative aging. The truth is that cavities can absolutely be avoided. Early childhood dental filling and drilling does not stop tooth decay; it only plugs the problem rather than getting to the root of the issue. The symptom is removed while the real issue—the cause of the decay—is overlooked.

At the age of eighteen months, teach your children to swish with salt water and to brush their teeth. Leave the toothbrush free of toothpaste. If a child's teeth are set close together, you, as the parent, will want to begin flossing them. It is easier than it sounds; rest the child's head on your lap to floss his teeth. Make it a fun family activity, and take your time. You are building a foundation for great oral health for a lifetime.

If a brown lesion appears on your child's tooth, keep it clean with salt rinses, baking soda, clay, and botanicals, while keeping your eye on it because it is still at a stage where the damage can be reversed. don't make the mistake of thinking that a lesion means you are on the road to a cavity. That may happen, but it is completely reversible. The dentine inside the tooth is sending out odontoblasts, new cellular growth, to the area. The tooth is healing itself. The brown area, when healed, will still have good strong enamel.

Bonding agents, or sealants, are often recommended by dentists to prevent cavities in children. To seal the teeth, the dentist etches the tooth and fills the micropores with a plastic resin, sealing the pits and fissures of the teeth, which are often sites for decay. This seems like a practical intervention, but sealants leak a toxic plastic chemical called bisphenol A, otherwise known as BPA, and the seal only lasts about a year. Sealants are not removed, so where do they go? The procedure may protect the teeth from bacteria, but some bacteria are trapped underneath the sealant, leaving the tooth even weaker when the sealant is gone. A new technique has been developed to prevent bacteria getting trapped underneath the sealant; the tooth is cleaned with a drill burr, removing part of the tooth. In the end, the child is ultimately left with a tiny filling on a new, healthy tooth to prevent the need for a cavity filling. How can this make sense?

Chapter 6

Braces: Integrated Health or Heavy Metal

Today's teenagers view getting braces as a rite of passage. When you were ten years old, you were dragged into an orthodontist's office and left with a mouth full of metal braces, brackets, wires, and bands to straighten your teeth after a few hours of fitting, gluing, and tapping. To allow for appropriately spaced teeth in your mouth, it's possible that some of your permanent teeth were extracted beforehand.

In medicine, crowded teeth are referred to as malocclusion, or "bad bite." The majority of Western children nowadays suffer from malocclusion, which is characterized by an overbite, underbite, or crooked teeth, and as a result, they spend years having ceramic, titanium, nickel, and stainless-steel veneers placed on their teeth. Modern malocclusion has a history; a few hundred years ago, crooked teeth were an unusual disaster, and a nasty bite was extremely uncommon a millennium ago.

Braces Alter Faces

A growing number of people use braces to straighten their teeth. In the United States, about four million people wear braces to address malocclusions on any given day. Although improving one's appearance is not the only objective of orthodontic treatment, wearing braces can be uncomfortable for some people. Even though someone has perfectly straight teeth after receiving braces, attractive appearances are about more than just well-aligned teeth. We could be misled into believing that orthodontic intervention is a risk-free panacea due to the widespread usage of braces. Orthodontists are better at this; often, before fitting someone for braces, they need a signed waiver-release form. These waivers describe the possible problems and hazards associated with braces and contain the following statements:

- As a living organism, your mouth's reaction to medical care cannot always be predicted.
- The objectives of treatment may be compromised by growth patterns that have an unforeseen impact on the teeth and facial tissues.
- Treatment may be hampered by unusual jaw growth and atypical tooth formation.
- Throughout life, the mouth is a dynamic system that adapts and changes. Following orthodontic treatment, modifications to the jaws, teeth, and face bones may have an impact on how teeth align.
- Braces work by applying forces to the teeth that cause cellular responses in the gums, surrounding tissues, and tooth roots. This allows the teeth to be moved and adjusted.

It is possible that these stresses will cause the nerves in a tooth to die.
- Braces have the potential to erode dental enamel and irreversibly harm tooth roots, which would jeopardize the teeth's viability.
- Brace-altered teeth may be more vulnerable to harm or even loss in the event of a gum or jaw accident in the future.

Scientific justification warrants these statements. It is important to understand the implications, because braces may be a detriment to your health and appearance. Research reported in the American Journal of Orthodontics and Dentofacial Orthopedics has shown that the tweaking and torquing of braces on teeth damages and shortens the roots of the teeth. A study that showed that fixed appliances like braces can damage enamel up to ninety percent of the time occurs soon after they are applied. This study was published in the same journal.

Enamel and roots can sustain irreversible damage. Conventional orthodontics may permanently damage a person's facial look, especially in children. Braces intentionally restrict or reroute the jaw's natural growth direction, which is normal. For instance, braces are used to correct an overbite by pulling back the upper jaw, which stunts natural growth. As a result, the face grows excessively vertically, or long, rather than normally.

Teeth Pulling

In orthodontic treatment, it is typical practice to extract the wisdom teeth and up to four teeth before using braces to create adequate room in the mouth for the braces to function. As omnivores, humans need jaws large enough to accommodate all thirty-two permanent teeth, but most orthodontists are taught that the size of our facial bones is an inherited genetic trait, and their treatment plan reflects this belief. If genetics determines that your jaw is too small for a full, straight set of permanent teeth, then some of your teeth must go. In addition to forming an expressive, ten-tooth smile, each tooth plays a part in the proper alignment of the cranial and facial bones and the effective metabolism of food. The symmetry, form, and overall youthful aspect of the face are all compromised when permanent teeth are removed. A longer, less full face with lower cheek bones, thinner lips, and an out-of-proportion nose are the aesthetic alterations that follow extractions, and they are comparable to the changes in the face that come with aging. A face that is noticeably out of proportion is frequently the outcome when these modifications are combined with the vertical development that braces promote.

For kids who are still developing and growing, extraction can be especially difficult. "Extracting teeth from children can result in less-than-optimal facial aesthetics," warns the Metal Mouth

Forum, a public forum on braces. In other words, instead of growing larger, your child's face may end up looking longer and fatter than it could have. Recognizing the vertical development trend brought on by orthodontia, an orthodontic publication carried out an experiment in which panel members evaluated the facial profiles of individuals to determine their attractiveness. Longer profiles are viewed as less attractive, the panel concluded.

Be Aware of Your Mouth

We must always breathe via our noses. Eventually, we may start breathing via our mouths due to a range of environmental factors. Particularly in early life, a mouth that is always hanging open to take in air alters craniofacial development. Children who breathe through their mouths have malocclusion and a vertical growth pattern in their faces, as a result of the deep, narrow form taken on by the roofs of their mouths and possible pulling back and down of the lower jaw. Furthermore, a wide palate is not formed when the tongue is not in the roof of the mouth long enough. A basic breathing therapy technique is the Buteyko method. This method can help you retrain your nose to breathe naturally if you or your child does.

As living structures, our teeth and face bones maintain their flexibility and health over the course of our lifetimes. Get multiple opinions and thoroughly weigh all of your alternatives, including functional orthodontia, before getting braces for yourself or your kids. Find out from the orthodontist how the braces and other treatments could enhance or detract from the beauty of your face. To witness the transformation for yourself, ask for before and subsequent profile photos of previous clients. You can discover a functional orthodontist by contacting the International Association of Facial Growth Guidance (www.orthotropics.com) or the

International Association for Orthodontics (www.iaortho.org).

We can help our children and future generations grow beautiful faces with plenty of room for a full set of evenly aligned teeth, and we might be able to completely avoid braces and orthodontic treatment if we give our bodies the nutrition they need to thrive. We should reconsider what constitutes the ideal smile as well. Accept the true beauty of your own smile and your children's grins, and release yourself and your kids from the prefabricated standard of beauty propagated by "beauty" magazines.

Chapter 7

Eight Steps to Self-Dentistry

The Effectiveness of the Successful Self-Dentistry routine in avoiding decay, bleeding gums, inflammation, and even colds will astound you if you follow it religiously.

These procedures should ideally be finished both morning and night because plaque starts to regenerate six hours after brushing. Gum tissue alerts your immune system to an issue after two to four days of non-compliance, and your immune system responds by deploying white blood cells to assist. The collagen strands that hold teeth to the jawbone break down as a result of this. Bacterial colonies are formed by biofilm within a week or two of neglect. At this point, bleeding gums are possible, especially after flossing.

Your teeth will feel as smooth and clean every day as if you've just returned from a dental hygienist's appointment thanks to the Successful Self-Dentistry routine, which will maintain your mouth, teeth, gums, and saliva in such perfect condition.

Step 1: The Salt-Water Rinse

Since most people have salt in their homes, you may get started on this practical step right now. Brushing in a neutral environment is made possible by salt, which also kills bacteria and raises the pH of the mouth to an alkaline level. When it's not the best time to brush your teeth, a salt rinse can help. Neutralizing the acidity as soon as possible after consuming citrus or other high-acid foods is very crucial.

Buy a shot glass and a Mason jar with a tight-fitting lid for every member of your family. Combine one ounce of salt with sixteen ounces of hot (nearly boiling) Springwater or unchlorinated, nonfluorinated water. The salt in the brine is activated and dissolved by the hot water. You can add a drop of essential oil to your brine and shake it, rather than stir it. Pour yourself a shot glass of the mixture, swish it around, spit, and repeat to use the saltwater rinse.

Step 2: Tongue Scraping

Bid farewell to morning breath: mucus and many bacteria from the alimentary canal migrate up onto the tongue's coating, especially during night. By carefully removing the covering, tongue scraping enhances dental health in general. It will also make your breath sweeter and food taste better. Better nourishment will mean that you have less scraping to do.

A spoon edge can be used, or you can get a tongue scraper from any health food store. The plaque will be erased if you only scrape your tongue from back to front. Once your tongue is clean, which should take two or three scrapes, rinse the scraper under hot water. Additionally, you can fill the scraper with one drop of a combination serum or essential oil.

Step 3: Brush the Gums

Pay close attention to this since it is highly crucial. For this phase, use a dry, manual toothbrush with soft bristles. Always brush the gums in the direction of the teeth, applying additional gentle pressure over the gum line, which is the point where the teeth and gums meet. Put a small amount of neem oil onto your dry toothbrush along with a drop of an essential oil or combo serum. As you move the brush from the gums toward the teeth, it should go upward for the bottom teeth and downward for the upper teeth. As carefully as possible, brush.

Give this step some careful thought. Relax by taking a seat on the toilet seat or the bathtub edge. Even better, you can brush with a pal outside. Have fun with it! The days of foamy sodium laurel sulfate mouthfuls and standing over the sink with the water flowing are long gone. I use my preferred light-activated ionic toothbrush at this time. By generating negative ions in the saliva, this brush removes 40% of plaque. The amount of plaque in the mouth is significantly reduced just by ionizing and alkalinizing the saliva.

Step 4: Teeth Polishing

In addition to giving, you smooth, silky teeth that you will love sliding your tongue over, polishing the teeth guarantees that any remaining plaque and discoloration are gone.

Best is an electric brush with a circular head. Having used a wide range of electric brushes, I believe that cheap rechargeable brushes work incredibly well. Areas inaccessible to a human brush are effortlessly cleaned with little round-headed electric brushes. Using a brush, apply a small amount of tooth polish, one drop of essential oil, or a combination serum, and brush over your teeth. Avoid the gums and concentrate just on the teeth. Mix equal parts baking soda and salt to create a highly powerful DIY tooth polish. In a minute or two, the biofilm and sticky plaque will be eliminated.

Step 5: Examine the Gum Lines

Due of the close correlation between gum health and tooth health, this step is immensely significant. Teeth are maintained robust and in their proper position by the gums. It's important to take proper care of the gums because they host thousands of microscopic filaments that connect the tooth to the jaw.

Using your tongue, feel for rough areas where plaque has accumulated along the inner and outer gum lines. Plaque frequently develops near the sulcus, or gum line, of the teeth. For this area, sulcus brushes and gum instruments with rubber tips are available. Using either tool, lightly apply a drop of essential oil or combination serum along the gum line on the inner and outside of each tooth.

Step 6: Flossing

As part of a heart-healthy lifestyle, think about flossing. If you detest flossing, you are about to experience a delightful revelation: adding essential oil to the floss makes it enjoyable and revitalizing. The strong plant oils are effectively cleansing your teeth. You will like flossing even more if you already enjoy it.

Pull out a lengthy floss strand. To coat the floss with essential oil, place one drop on your index finger and rub it between your thumb and index finger. Grasp the floss between your fingers and move it up, down, and back and forth in between your teeth. Make careful to floss the areas where food and plaque accumulate—the spaces between teeth and the area surrounding their necks.

Step 7: Final Rinse

You can also alternate mouth rinses: swish and rinse with one more shot of your handy-dandy mouth-rinse brine; swish, swish, swish, and spit;

the salt water and essential oils will coat your entire mouth, preventing the formation of bacteria and nourishing the tissue.

Step 8: Extra Gum Care

An oral irrigator, which is a syringe with a blunt end, is required for this procedure. Flossing, brushing, and scraping are unable to reach areas that are not reachable by the VitaPick brand of irrigator, which functions similarly to a tiny showerhead and flushes out the gum line. It will rinse out the microorganisms that you might have missed in earlier steps, and this irrigator has a finer spray than a Waterpick.

To fill your shot glass, add a drop or two of essential oil and a tiny quantity of your homemade saltwater mouthwash. The mixture from the shot glass should be drawn up into the syringe to fill the irrigator. Afterwards, clean each tooth's sulci and interstices, paying particular attention to any regions that require it. By doing so, the gum tissue will be revitalized and any leftover biofilms and bacteria will be destroyed. To relieve gum discomfort, strengthen antimicrobial defense, and improve breath, apply a few more drops of the oil to your gums.

Eight easy stages sum up the protocol. If you don't have the other ingredients on hand, you can start with simply salt and baking soda right immediately. Your oral ecology will noticeably improve if you adhere to these instructions on a daily basis—ideally twice a day.

Review of the Eight Steps
1. Maintain a saltwater solution near your teeth-brushing station. Add a drop of a combination serum or essential oil. Rinse with saltwater first, then brush.
2. Make two or three scrapes on the tongue.
3. Brush the gums, being very cautious around the gum line and mindful to brush from the gums toward the teeth.

Apply a tiny drop of neem oil together with a drop of an essential oil or combo serum using a gentle, dry brush.

4. Using an electric toothbrush with a round head that is dry, buff your teeth. Mix a small amount of homemade tooth polish with a drop of essential oil.

5. With a drop of an essential oil or combination serum, use a rubber-tipped gum tool or sulcus brush to remove any leftover plaque from the gum lines.

6. Floss! Better yet, floss twice. Put a drop of a combination serum or essential oil on the floss.

7. Use mouthwash or other rinses instead of salt. Give it a forceful swish and then spit.

8. Rinse the gum pockets with salt water and essential oil using the oral irrigator. Apply a small amount of oil or serum to the gum line and other delicate regions.

Chapter 8

Botanicals that are Beneficial

The best ally for our well-being is nature. For millennia, therapeutic uses have made use of plant, flower, seed, root, and tree distillations. Botanical oils, which comprise essential oils and supercritical extracts, provide us with gentle, effective, and safe support and protection from head to toe.

Because all botanical oils have antibacterial, antifungal, and antiviral properties, they eliminate undesirable mouth germs. Through the renewal of gum tissue and the enhancement of blood circulation to the gums and blood vessels of the mouth, they optimize the well-being of our oral environment. They deal with the conditions that cause a weakened immune system, such as pathogens, viruses, long-term inflammation, and a clogged lymphatic system. Because essential plant extracts provide pharmacological effects, the use of authentic essential oils began as a kind of medicinal therapy. Unfortunately, the usage of essential oils for aromatherapy has been consigned to the trivial world of potpourri and perfumery due to the current commercialization and creation of synthetic flavors and perfumes.

Unlike herbal tinctures, homeopathic medicines, or dietary supplements, these unique plant extracts are not the same. They are the concentrated forms of the plants that go by those names. The integrity of hundreds of plant-derived botanical chemicals as well as trace elements referred to as secondary metabolites are preserved in each genuine essence through gradual, low-temperature distillation. The plant's adaptogens, or secondary metabolites, are distinct from the plant's DNA and basic structure. The aromatic hormones, phenols, and pheromones that draw pollinators, ward off insects, and contribute to the distinctive individual expression of the plant are these adaptogen compounds. These plant materials' components closely resemble the hormones, enzymes, and neurotransmitters found in humans, thereby elegantly illustrating the biological harmony that exists between humans and plants. Their strong impact on our well-being is made possible by their biocompatibility.

Highly concentrated lipophilic liquids are essential oils and supercritical extracts. An entire plant or more is needed to produce a single drop of oil for some of the botanical oils. Oils are incredibly powerful, frequently hundreds of times more potent than the herbal extract, and they contain countless beneficial chemical components that interact harmoniously with our bodies and each other. Essential oils can swiftly reach the immune system because of their unique lipid-soluble nature, which enables them to pass through the lipid layer of our skin and gums. A favorable mosaic effect is produced when hundreds of plant components, some of which are antibacterial, some of which are analgesic, and some of which reduce inflammation, are mixed with botanical oils.

The gums' lipid matrix is easily penetrated by all essential oils and supercritical extracts. The blood vessels, dentine, nerves, and tooth roots all receive nutrients from them. They initiate the oral and lymphatic systems and promote circulation. Gum tissue can regenerate with the aid of certain oils, including those found in sea buckthorn berries. Additionally, they have a strong capability for oxygen radical absorbance (ORAC). Cinnamon and cloves have remarkable antibacterial qualities and are also quite high in ORAC.

Pure aromatic molecules have a direct pathway through the blood-brain barrier into the hypothalamus, the center of the mind. Once inside the hypothalamus, the brain releases neurotransmitters, including encephalin, endorphins, serotonin, and noradrenalin. Endorphins and encephalins reduce pain and produce a pleasant, euphoric state of mind and feelings of well-being. Serotonin is calming and relaxing. Noradrenalin is stimulating and maintains mental clarity.

My go-to botanical for strong teeth and gums is a combination serum made from the supercritical extracts and essences of tea tree, cinnamon, thyme linalool, rose otto, oregano, peppermint, clove, and sea-buckthorn berry. In addition, I prepare a potent botanical combination serum based on ancient Vedic principles, combining extracts of neem, cinnamon, clove, cayenne, mastic, and cardamom.

As your body's intuition develops and leads you to the ideal oils or blends for you, you might wish to try a few single essential oils. I'm sure you want to be sure anything is genuine and pure before putting it on your body, in your mouth, or in your child's mouth. Market-available essential oils, even those found in health food stores, are frequently of dubious quality. These oils are cheaply made, further contaminated in labs, and may even be imitations. They are mass-distilled for the food, fragrance, and beauty sectors. Low-quality essential oils have safety and efficacy concerns, thus using them is not advised. The promises of plant wisdom can only be fulfilled by genuine oils that are properly and honestly distilled from organically grown plant matter.

These botanical oils are some of the greatest for promoting dental health at its best.

- **Cardamom (Elettaria cardamomum):** In addition to its antibacterial qualities, which boost the immune system's phagocytic cellular activity, this essential oil activates and tones the digestive tract. In addition to its anti-infective and antibacterial properties, it supports the nervous system and contributes to good dental hygiene.

- **Cayenne (Capsicum Frutescens):** Pick a supercritical extract that has stimulating, catalytic, antiseptic, and antibacterial qualities. Additionally, a topical vasodilator that promotes blood circulation is the capsaicin component found in cayenne. In order to use it, dilute it first.

- **Cinnamon (Cinnamomum Ceylanicum):** Antiseptic and antibacterial, genuine cinnamon-bark essential oil is native to Sri Lanka and the Malabar Coast of India. It encourages blood flow to the gums, which in turn supports gum health and regeneration. Strong analgesic and antiseptic qualities found in cinnamon, along with a high concentration of cineole and eugenol, stimulate the development of white blood cells. Ninety-eight percent of all pathogenic microorganisms can be defeated by cinnamon bark oil. Since this oil is highly potent, it must be diluted before using.

- **Clove bud (Eugenia Caryophyllata):** With a very high ORAC, clove oil is an analgesic that is extracted from the clove tree's blossoming buds. Since ancient times, cloves have helped with toothaches and breath freshening. Clove is a powerful antibacterial, antiviral, and antifungal that also stimulates blood flow and strengthens the immune system. Its botanical constituents, eugenol, esters, and sesquiterpenes, work together to create an impressive action against microbes and pathogens. Clove is also antiparasitic and helps with gum infections, toothaches, and tonsillitis. Before using clove oil, dilute it.

- **Oregano (Origanum vulgare):** Wild oregano oil, which is gathered from the mountains surrounding the Mediterranean, offers a wide range of botanical advantages. It is approximately 65 percent carvacrol and 3.4 percent thymol, two phenol constituents that add to its therapeutic efficacy. These phenols have strong analgesic, antibacterial, and antiseptic qualities. Oregano boosts the immune system and functions essentially like an antibiotic. A wide variety of bacteria, viruses, and fungi, such as E. Coli, Staphylococcus aureus, and Pseudomonas aeruginosa, can be effectively combated by oregano. By eliminating plaque-causing germs and lowering the risk of gum disease, wild oregano oil can enhance dental hygiene when applied topically. You have to dilute oregano oil before using it.

- **Peppermint (Mentha piperita):** Mint contains anti-inflammatory, analgesic, and cooling properties in addition to aiding with digestion. Peppermint oil use prevents radiation-induced glutathione reductions and lowers oxidized fat levels in bodily tissue. There are many places to buy peppermint oil, but if you want the purest, most potent oil, go for a real distillation made from fresh peppermint leaves cultivated in France. It's critical to realize that commercial toothpaste contains artificial menthol, which tastes like peppermint and has no real value in avoiding gingivitis. True peppermint reduces teeth decay-causing germs and is a powerful antioxidant.
- **Tea tree oil (Melaleuca alternifolia):** Originating from the paper bark tea tree, native Australians have been using tea as a medicinal herb for thousands of years. It

resists viruses, fungi, and bacteria. According to the Australian Dental Journal, it is used as a treatment agent for illnesses including periodontitis and persistent gingivitis, which are characterized by inflammation and germs. Tea tree contains plant compounds called cineol and propanol that have anti-inflammatory properties and can help reduce plaque and gingivitis. In addition, tea tree is highly antibacterial and astringent.

- **Thyme linalool (Thymus ct linalool):** This particular kind of thyme is uncommon. It has a mild yet antibacterial quality, balances salivary secretions in the mouth, boosts immunity, and decongestant properties. As an immunostimulant with antimicrobial medicines, it is generally tonifying and effective.

Despite having distinct synergy, all of the botanical oils and combination serums that I suggest provide the same outstanding outcomes. They work wonders for brushing, flossing, and maintaining healthy gums. They affect the entire body in addition to keeping your mouth healthy. Therefore, the botanicals and serums are a part of a holistic, harmonic system that helps your entire body, even if your attention is solely on your teeth and gums.

It is a common question to know if it is safe to ingest supercritical extracts and essential oils. In the droplet amounts that they are used in, it is safe to consume them. Because essential oils are powerful, labels at health food stores frequently state that taking them internally in any amount is unsafe. This is applicable to oils that lack a true, organic, and authentic distillation. Nonetheless, the majority of pure essential oil distillations are safe and frequently advantageous for internal use when consumed in modest doses, typically one drop. In actuality, the food and cosmetics sectors use a lot of essential oils. Essential oils derived from oranges are often used for orange juice, while bergamot essential oil is preferred for Earl Grey tea. A variety of essential oils are also used in liqueurs, confections, chocolates, and favor extracts.

Chapter 9

Extra Tooth Tips

Preserving Alkaline Bodies

Litmus paper is that yellow strip of paper you played with in science class; you can use it to evaluate the alkalinity of your urine and saliva. To get the body to become alkaline, one must eat a nutritious, healthful diet. Alkalinizing meals include baking soda, magnesium, and greens such as spirulina, chlorella, and smoothies made with vegetables.

Atomic Mouth Gargle with Iodine

Use iodine in its atomic form to make an immune-boosting mouth mouthwash. Rapid bactericidal action, relief from oral thrush, and thyroid gland support are all provided by atomic iodine. Either once a week or every other day, just add one drop to a glass of water to drink.

Baking Soda

I used to believe that sodium bicarbonate, or baking soda, was this weird white powder. I now realize that sodium bicarbonate is a crucial component found in all body fluids and organs. It is essential for digestion and is contained in saliva, which is generated by our stomachs. It is completely safe to use baking soda devoid of aluminum to clean teeth, and it can even be used as a supplement to keep pH levels stable. Bacterial acidity is neutralized by the inherent alkalinity of baking soda. By increasing calcium intake to the enamel, preventing dental caries, reducing dental plaque, and counteracting the effects of damaging metabolic acids, it is a buffer.

For ages, people have used baking soda as toothpaste, frequently in combination with sea salt. Baking soda is not only a mild cleaning agent but also quite effective. Compared to the cleansing ingredients in the majority of commercial toothpastes, such as silica and chalk, it is much less abrasive. Destructive gum disease can be avoided by regularly brushing your teeth with baking soda and salt.

The preventative benefits of baking soda are widely praised by dentists, and now is a great time to incorporate this magic ingredient into your oral hygiene routine.

Blood Tests

A valuable diagnostic method for oral and systemic health issues is blood testing. Acquiring the appropriate expert or physician to evaluate the findings is the tricky part. The tests I suggest are as follows:

- **Hormone panel:** Men and women are examined for distinct hormones. Progesterone levels should be measured in menstruating women between days 18 and 22 of their cycle.

- **C-reactive protein (CRP) and homocysteine levels:** This will examine the indicators to see if the body has any systemic inflammation. They serve as excellent overall health markers.
- **Complete blood count:** See how the dental material and immune system are getting along by running a complete blood count (CBC) before and after major dental treatments.
- **Thyroid:** TSH levels, or thyroid-stimulating hormone.
- **General vitamins and minerals test:** Inspect the body's nutrient absorption capacity and look for any nutritional inadequacies.
- **Blood sugar:** You are able to check your own blood sugar levels. You can buy a monitor at any pharmacy. Every

morning, check your blood sugar level after a fast.

Breath

There are undoubtedly a lot of advertisements concerning halitosis, or bad breath. If your breath seems less than fresh after brushing and flossing and you do not have any cavities, beyond the foul breath induced by eating garlic or light plaque, this could be your body's way of telling you that something needs to be adjusted. Your body might be handling a high number of bacteria as a result of an infection, or you might experience dry mouth at night from medicine, sleep apnea, or snoring-related reduced salivary flow. Digging further and looking into stomach problems can also be necessary. The intestinal tract's health is reflected in the state of the mouth. The main reasons of bad breath may include gas, bloating, constipation, sulfur compounds expelled from the stomach, and elevated blood sugar levels.

Make sure there is no active decay in the mouth, like as problems with root canals or decay beneath a crown filling, in order to treat halitosis. Twice daily, follow the Eight Steps. Examine your digestive system to see whether your body need clay therapy, probiotics, enzymes, or colonics in order to regain equilibrium.

Clay

Since ancient times, clay has been utilized for both exterior and internal cleaning. Clay can be used topically or soaked in to pull toxins and heavy metals out of the body through the skin. Another way that ingesting clay works is by drawing toxins out of the mouth and digestive system. Clay operates in a dynamic state of ionic exchange with the alimentary canal during bodily interactions. It takes up positively charged pollutants and toxins, leaving behind negatively charged nutrients that are good for you.

Another great material for teeth brushing is clay. To remove plaque from your toothbrush, just sprinkle extremely fine powdered clay—

bentonite, zeolite, or silica-rich clay—onto it when it's dry. Cleansing clay baths are another gentle method of detoxification. To improve your bathing experience, add a drop of the immune-boosting, lymph-stimulating essential oils of juniper, grapefruit, and cypress along with baking soda and clays to your warm water bath.

Dry Brushing

Dry brushing is a fantastic longevity practice that stimulates the lymphatic system before regular baths, showers, or saunas.

Handling Severe Gum inflammation

Huggins gives this advice in the Eight Steps, but it is so useful that I am giving it again here. For the first two days, treat inflamed gums by putting half a teaspoon of purified salt in a glass of hot water and swishing it around in your mouth roughly every hour. Rinse with sodium ascorbate vitamin C powder that has been dissolved in hot water after 30 minutes.

Healing Herbs

The tea that is brewed from little tea bags is not the same as herbal tea. Make a large pot of tea to sip throughout the day instead of brewing just a little cup with a teabag as we have done in the past. One of my favorite ways to make herbal tea is to fill a quart-sized Mason jar with one or two ounces of dry herbs. Pour in nearly boiling water, cover the jar, and leave it to steep for the entire night. After the herbs are strained, sip. After giving them an overnight soak, you can fill multiple jars in this way and store them in the refrigerator.

I suggest toning the liver, skin, and digestive system with a mineral-rich tea made with horsetail, nettles, and dandelion. It also fortifies gums and dental enamel. Horsetail contains a high silica content, nettles are abundant in calcium and iron, and dandelion helps strengthen teeth.

Herbs can also be added to your mouthwash made with saltwater. Use ginger, mullein, goldenseal, grape root, or white oak bark. Your teeth and gums will receive a spa treatment from an herbal powder poultice; it's like a tiny face mask for your mouth. Take one capsule or a dash of powdered white oak bark, astragalus, or goldenseal, and then blend in a drop of essential oil or combination serum until a paste forms. Then, fill the spaces between your teeth and the regions that require more attention with this mixture. You can also mix the plants with clay.

Detox for Heavy Metal

Toxic chemicals known as heavy metals can build up in body fat and the blood. Numerous harmful wastes have been deposited into our bodies throughout decades of industrialization. To gently chelate the body using a combination of herbs, vitamins, and therapies, a multimodal approach works best. A heavy metal detox can also be achieved by regular sauna sweats and dry brushing, or by scheduling several colonics once or twice a year. In addition, it's essential to throw out all synthetic cleaning supplies and body care "beauty" items in order to become and remain clean.

Additionally, you should take superoxide dismutase (SOD), milk thistle, glutathione, turmeric, and natural B vitamins to promote liver function. Maintaining a healthy flow of evacuation is essential to prevent stagnation and reabsorption. To aid in the detoxification of your bowels, soak a teaspoon of bentonite clay in a glass of water overnight and drink the mixture first thing in the morning. You can also take a tablespoon of chia seeds.

Homeopathy

Homeopathic medicines employ extremely diluted chemicals according to the "like cures like" theory. For instance, tiny amounts of homeopathic Rhus toxin, also referred to as poison ivy, can stop and treat the plant's itchy allergic reaction. These treatments strengthen, cleanse, and address the underlying causes of oral imbalances, making them helpful instruments for maintaining a balanced oral ecology. Certain biological dentists, including as Dr. Gerald Smith, who employs RIFE technology in conjunction with German Sanum brand remedies, inject homeopathic remedies into extraction sites to treat the side effects of cavities, root canals, and imbalances in the saliva and enamel. "If you hit the right remedy for the right problem, it will work through mint, coffee, alcohol, or anything else," claims Smith. The following are only a few suggestions from the extensive field of homeopathic therapy. See the "Resources" guide at the conclusion of the book for more detailed information, or speak with a homeopath.

- Belladonna is useful in treating TMJ disorders and abscesses.

- Hypericum is used to heal bacterially damaged tissue.
- Arnica is used to treat dental work, injuries to the teeth, extractions, and swelling-related discomfort.
- The best toothache cure is Plantago.
- Strong toothaches that drive you "crazy" should be treated with coffee.

Salts from Tissue and Cells

These salts are an additional application of homeopathy, created by German physician Dr. Wilhelm Heinrich Schussler, that is based on inorganic mineral salts. These are some options we have for cell salts that you could use in your dental apothecary:

- **Calc fluor:** Recommended for weak tissue elasticity, sensitive teeth, decay, and poor tooth enamel. I can personally attest to the efficacy of calc fluor. I found out after a few ardent weeks of eating fresh wild bee pollen that it had damaged my teeth enamel since it was slightly acidic. Fortunately, I happened to run into my friend who is a naturopathic doctor, and she told me about her experience. She suggested swishing with water and three or four calc fluor cell salt pills. I'm pleased to say that after three days, my enamel returned to normal.

- **Calc Phos:** could aid in bringing the ratios of calcium to phosphorus in the bones into equilibrium. Building strong dentine and enamel is its main purpose. Additionally, it is mixed with calcium fluoride to treat decay and as a teething treatment. Regard the internal tooth matrix as Calc Phos and the external tooth matrix as calc fluor.

- **Nat Mur (sodium chloride):** It regulates the flow of water into and out of the cells to keep the body's water balance stable. Recommended for cracked tongue, dry mouth, and cold sores.

- **Silica:** Blood, skin, hair, nails, bones, nerve sheaths, and some tissues all contain significant amounts of it. When pus forms in abscesses, pus pockets, or gum infections, it is a beneficial treatment.

Hydrogen Peroxide

Food-grade hydrogen peroxide should be on hand. It must be diluted to a concentration of three percent before to usage because it is extremely potent and undiluted. The best way to clean dental instruments and toothbrushes is with peroxide. Every family member's toothbrush can be kept overnight in a little glass filled with a solution of three percent hydrogen peroxide. Do not forget to alter the solution every day.

Once a year, hydrogen peroxide can be used to remove stains from teeth or occasionally to clean up a gum pocket. Rinse with salt water right away in order to neutralize and alkalinize. Using it on a daily basis is too harsh on the gums and enamel, and excessive use might cause your gums to recede.

Magnesium Oil Cleansing

In its pure, natural form, magnesium chloride helps strengthen and repair teeth and tissue. Magnesium is a necessary mineral for the bone matrix and for the correct absorption of calcium needed to create strong enamel. Another great mouthwash for restoring oral ecology is a natural liquid magnesium chloride solution. It is possible to ingest the purest form. Depending on your oral health, use the mouthwash at full strength or dilute it up to 50%. Use it once a day or once a week. For children's use, dilute it.

Therapy with Oil Pulling

An age-old Ayurvedic practice called oil pulling is used to treat bleeding gums, whiten teeth, and improve bad breath. Mix one drop of oregano essential oil, one drop of organic virgin coconut oil or olive oil, and one drop of another essential oil or combo serum to rinse the mouth. After 10 minutes of rapidly swishing this combination around the mouth, spit it out. Toxins are drawn out of teeth and gums by the oil.

Ozone Therapy for Dental Health

Ozone treatment was created by the clever and imaginative Nikola Tesla. Being an electrical genius, he received over three hundred patents covering topics such as wireless communication, ionized gases, cold plasma, and wireless lightbulbs. Tesla received a patent for an ozone generator in 1896. He started the Tesla Ozone Company and used ozone to bubble olive oil until a potent gel hardened, suitable for use by naturopaths and physicians.

Three oxygen atoms make up the chemical known as ozone (O3), which has inherent antiviral, antifungal, and antibacterial properties. Ozone is now employed in biological dentistry procedures as ozone gas and ozone-infused water. Ozone is useful in dentistry in numerous ways:

- It is injected all the way around a tooth that has a root canal.
- Ozone gas exposure causes cavities to harden.
- When a nerve is exposed, ozone gas and water combined will frequently stop the nerve from dying.
- Applying ozone water irrigation to a surgical site can hasten the healing process and promote bone remineralization.
- A step in the cavitation removal technique involves injecting ozone gas into the affected area.

- Ozone injections into the TMJ joint have been shown to have anti-inflammatory properties.
- Gum pockets can be irrigated, gargled, and consumed with ozonated water.

To provide the combined benefits of ozone and powerful botanicals at home, there are also ozonated tooth serums available. Gums, sensitive teeth, abscesses, gum pockets, sulci, oral lesions, and cold sores can all be treated with these ozonated serums.

Salt

An easy-to-use yet effective alkalinizing and antibacterial agent is salt. Huggins advises against using sea salt since it contains nonbiological potassium and is frequently tainted with lead, mercury, cadmium, and other heavy metals. Instead, he suggests using only pure sodium chloride (purified salt). Moreover, sea salt no longer has its inherent electrical charge. The body's cells engage in a significant electrical exchange that involves the elements sodium, potassium, and chloride. To replenish the sodium and potassium's electron stores, dissolve the salt in boiling water.

Saunas

Heaters for far-infrared saunas liberate heavy metals through the body's glands by emitting a certain wavelength. Sweating is a safe and efficient method of eliminating accumulated toxins since it excretes them through the skin as opposed to the liver and kidneys, which are burdened by labor.

Thyroid Care

The thyroid is ineffective in a lot of people. Everyday occurrences such as radiation, heavy metals, and BPA seeping from food containers and plastic fillings have a significant impact on the thyroid gland. Fluoride in toothpaste and water, brominated food, and chlorine showers are its burdens. Mercury poisoning, even at low concentrations, can disrupt cell division, leading to exhaustion and a drop in body temperature, which further complicates the thyroid's ability to maintain homeostasis. Thyroid-stimulating hormone (TSH) levels in the blood may indicate a heavy metal issue if they are more than 2 milli-IU per liter.

Toothaches

Think of a toothache is your mouth's alarm. Bacteria piercing both the nerve and the enamel could be the culprit, or it could be a damaged nerve. Dilute organic clove or rose otto essential oil in organic olive oil, virgin coconut oil, or your preferred essential oil serum for an antimicrobial and analgesic first aid therapy. Every 30 minutes, apply it to the afflicted area until the discomfort subsides. Another choice is to use a VitaPick irrigator or a blunt-tipped syringe to inject the rose or clove oil into the gum line or affected area after diluting it 1:3 with olive oil. Next, to produce a spotless, sealed space, coat the teeth with frankincense resin or propolis paste.

The immune system can be strengthened with additional vitamin C, reishi tincture, vitamin D, chaga tea, olive leaf extract, oil of oregano (dilute wild oregano essential oil to five percent with ninety-five percent olive oil), and pine bark extract to prevent toothaches from their underlying causes. Intriguingly, recent studies have also discovered that injectable methyl form of vitamin B12 helps improve unknown tooth pain and neuralgia associated with jaw infection.

The Temporomandibular Joints
On the left and right sides of the face, the temporomandibular joints (TMJs) connect the upper and lower jaw. More than 130 muscles are connected to the lower jaw. The occipital ridge, the neck, the shoulder girdle, and the teeth are all affected by these muscles and joints, which also have an impact on the pelvic girdle and a person's stride or gait. These muscles, along

with the upper and lower jaw, can be misaligned for a variety of reasons, such as forceps delivery during birth, fillings, root canals, extractions, and overuse of dental procedures, particularly when teeth have been ground down or eviscerated. Proprioception is the unconscious sense of movement and spatial orientation resulting from stimuli within the body itself. According to Nunnally, "teeth grinding and clenching are the main causes of receding gums." A clicking sound that you experience when you open and close your mouth could mean that your TMJ needs to be realigned and balanced. Stress and headaches may result from compression in the joint brought on by an uneven bite. Because of TMJ issues, the muscles surrounding the eyes might tense up and shorten, which results in nearsightedness and impaired vision.

Water

Never stop drinking water! Constant dryness prevents saliva from doing its job of lubricating teeth. For your body, fresh Springwater is ideal. Though clean, reverse osmosis water can remove minerals from your body since it is depleted of vital minerals. Steer clear of tap water as fluoride and chlorine can be harmful to teeth. Find out whether there is a natural spring nearby that may be used for water collection by speaking with locals and visiting the spring database at www.findaspring.com.

Our bodies are amazingly well-designed. Our teeth are taken care of by an internal mechanism that is part of who we are. Our bodies can flourish if we remove anything that prevents them from doing their natural job. Our teeth react to our efforts, which makes external maintenance—brushing, flossing, and cleaning—so simple. The living nature of our teeth allows for their condition to change over time. Living tissue makes up the pulp, dentine, enamel, and gums, all of which can be reinforced, repaired, and renewed with careful care.

The End

www.ingramcontent.com/pod-product-compliance
Lightning Source LLC
Chambersburg PA
CBHW032210220526

45471CB00004B/1905